Fuel Fantastic Sugar Cleanse

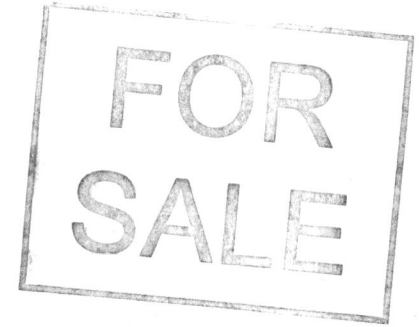

Fuel Fantastic Sugar Cleanse

Free Yourself of Sugar's Grasp in 21 Days or Less!

Kelly Fitzsimmons

Contents

Introduction

Throughout the guide, we interchangeably use the words 'sugar cleanse' and 'sugar detox'. For all intents and purposes, they are the exact same thing.

What you will find in this guide

- Detailed instructions on how to sugar cleanse
- Extra motivation to complete your cleanse
- Reasons why sugar is bad for your health
- Benefits of a sugar cleanse
- Healthy foods that are free of sugar
- Unhealthy foods that perpetuate poor health
- A Complete Shopping list
- Bonus chapters
- Sugar detox food pyramid
- Next steps…What to do after your 1st sugar cleanse.
- And more…

What you will not find in this guide

This guide is not meant to be a full fledge diet plan with its advice centered around losing weight, nutrition and effective exercises. A sugar cleanse is the ultimate precursor to making an easy transition to a permanent lifestyle change of eating clean, training mean and getting lean.

If you are looking for a sustainable, lifestyle plan, please refer to the original book in the Fuel Fantastic series.

Sugar is an 'Empty Calorie'

We've all heard this saying many, many times over. Usually the writer seems like they're on 'damage control' with their nutritional advice aimed at deflecting the negative media sugar receives on a daily basis.

This statement does much more harm than good. Yes, technically the statement is true but the nutritional picture it paints is very false.

If sugar receives bad press, it's for good reason.

- Sugar has no nutritional value. Meaning sugar actually deprives our bodies of the nutrients that is needed to process the sugar and sugar doesn't give anything back.
- Sugar is extremely stealthy and hides in all prepackaged and processed foods. All the natural flavors have been taken out and replaced with sugar to make the food palatable and tasty.
- Sugar also manages to sneak its way into most drinks, including fruit juices, sodas and sport drinks. Sugar also sneaks into most condiments and is now even found in baby formula.

Health Issues

- Simple sugars have been documented to cause and/or contribute to numerous health problems such as: mood disorders, asthma, nervous disorders, mental illness, heart disease, diabetes, gallstones, arthritis and hypertension.
- Cancer's favorite fuel is none other than sugar, glucose to be exact. Which is why managing your sugar intake is so

important to your health. Proper management can make a dramatic difference in cancer prevention and in cancer treatment.

- Glycation is partly to blame for sugar's health concerns. This process consists of the sugar in the blood attaching itself to proteins. This forms dangerous molecules known as 'advanced glycation end products.' As more and more of these are created, they start to damage the proteins nearby, in a domino effect. (see the Bonus Chapter: The Dangers of Glycation)
- Sugar also damages your skin by making it brittle and dry. This leads to sagging skin, wrinkles and leaves you more prone to sun damage and aging.

These are just a small sampling of the ill effects sugar causes to your health and diet.

My Personal Addiction to Sugar

My sugar addiction began at nine years old. Of course, at the time I didn't know it was going to become an addiction. My paper route allowed me to buy as much candy as my little heart desired and it turned out that my little heart desired more than my stomach could handle. Thus, my life of excess sugar consumption started very early on and in combination with my addictive personality, I always craved more.

After growing up, my tastes for sugar evolved multiple times and eventually I settled on soy vanilla lattes as my preferred craving. Honestly, I could never get enough of them!

This dark brown nectar of the gods always seemed to be the perfect combination of sweet and bitter. I also relished the epic caffeine boost that made me feel like the Energizer Bunny.

My morning latte allowed me to work like a mad man for the next hour or so, then just as suddenly as this boost occurred it stopped.

I crashed, bottomed out and it was a struggle just to look busy let alone get any meaningful work done. It felt like my body couldn't function without its next soy vanilla latte prescription. I had absolutely no energy to do anything.

At lunchtime, my body perked up at the thought of fulfilling my cravings with the enchanting potion. Somehow there was always just enough energy to crawl back to the coffee shop and buy another cup. And it was the most wonderful cup in the whole world, until the next one.

My life was revolving around all these sugary coffees. All they were doing was holding me back from living a real life. I started gaining weight and becoming even slower at work and in my other daily activities.

Then I realized this wasn't how I wanted to live. Quitting this lifestyle took all the energy and willpower I could muster and going it cold turkey was the only way I could do it.

Now years later, I feel better than I ever did! I have more energy, it's much easier to concentrate and my productivity is way up. It's even hard for me to slow down now and looking back I can't believe it took me so look to embrace this healthy lifestyle change.

I want everyone to know it is a challenge to overcome your sugar addiction, but it is possible and the results are completely worth it! My hope is my story and this guide will inspire you to live healthier and break free of sugar's grasp.

Medical Disclaimer

This book contains general information about diet and medical conditions. The information is not advice, and should not be treated as such.

The diet and medical information in this book are provided "as is" without any representations or warranties.

Kelly Quinn Fitzsimmons makes no representations or warranties in relation to the diet and medical information in this book.

You must not rely on the information in this book as an alternative to medical advice from your doctor or other professional healthcare provider.

If you have any specific questions about any medical matter you should consult your doctor or other professional healthcare provider.

If you think you may be suffering from any medical condition you should seek immediate medical attention.

You should never delay seeking medical advice, disregard medical advice, or discontinue medical treatment because of information in this book.

1

What is your Motivation to Sugar Detox?

Everyone has their own reason to complete a sugar detox. Maybe your reason is one of the following:

- you want to lose weight
- you want to correct chronic feelings of low energy
- you feel powerless to your sugar cravings
- you feel weak and sick all the time
- you desire more out of life
- you want to feel strong and vibrant
- your life seems to be stuck in a rut
- you have unexplained mood swings
- all of the above!

The Good News

The good news is, the longer you have sugar out of your system the less you will crave it. A detox doesn't need to be a permanent change in your diet but rather a re-setting of the way your body gets energy and a re-setting of the way it asks for this energy.

You'll begin to feel far more energetic as you won't be subjected to the energy highs and lows that sugar produces.

You will also notice other benefits, such as improved complexion and younger looking skin. This is because sugar consumption leads to the reduction of collagen in the skin.

I guess before you start, the question you need to ask yourself is whether or not you need to complete a sugar detox?

The Symptoms

Here are some of the things you can look for to alert yourself that your blood sugar levels might be out of balance:

- Tiredness after eating
- Needing caffeine for energy
- Cravings for sugar or bakery products
- Dizziness when missing meals
- Frequent hunger pangs
- Problems sleeping
- Continued cravings for sugar even after eating some
- Problems losing weight

Going through life with unbalanced blood sugar levels can lead to problems with insulin production and this may develop into more serious medical problems such as diabetes, metabolic syndrome and insulin resistance.

You might be very surprised to find out the true dangers of consuming a diet high in sugar and the detrimental damage it is doing to your health.

2

Fundamental Principles

The basic fundamental principles that guides people to cleanse their systems of sugar are:

- Sugar is Addictive
- Sugar Makes You Fat
- Sugar Causes Many Diseases

Trust me, there are many, many more reasons to detox but we wanted to keep this guide simple and concise; not long and boring.

Even if you decide not to cleanse your system of sugar, it would be beneficial for you to read the next three chapters and learn more about the dangers of excessive sugar consumption.

3

Sugar is Addictive

Nowadays, sugar is everywhere and included in almost everything. Its addictive nature causes a perpetual cycle of energy ups and downs that the average person never escapes from.

SUGAR ADDICTION:
THE PERPETUAL CYCLE

1. YOU EAT SUGAR
- YOU LIKE IT, YOU CRAVE IT
- IT HAS ADDICTIVE PROPERTIES

2. BLOOD SUGAR LEVELS SPIKE
- DOPAMINE IS RELEASED IN THE BRAIN = ADDICTION
- MASS INSULIN SECRETED TO DROP BLOOD SUGAR LEVELS

3. BLOOD SUGAR LEVELS FALL RAPIDLY
- HIGH INSULIN LEVELS CAUSE IMMEDIATE FAT STORAGE
- BODY CRAVES THE LOST SUGAR 'HIGH'

4. HUNGER & CRAVINGS
- LOW BLOOD SUGAR LEVELS CAUSE INCREASED APPETITE AND CRAVINGS
- THUS THE CYCLE IS REPEATED

When you consume sugar, it stimulates the release of two neurotransmitters, dopamine and serotonin into the nucleus accumbens (located in the brain) giving you a feeling of pleasure and happiness. The nucleus accumbens is known to play a vital role in addiction, pleasure and placebo. Sugar feeds directly into this and begins your addiction.

According to a study[1] conducted by Colantuoni, too much sugar can lead to dependency and create withdrawal like symptoms. Consuming too much sugar can also lead to many other potential health problems, which you'll read about further on.

Sugar addiction is like any other addiction. First, cravings start small and slowly begin to increase over time.

Whenever sugar is consumed these cravings subside and your brain begins the chemical production of opioids and dopamine (chemicals that make you feel happy).

This is a crucial part in the sugar high.

The next sensation you experience is a sudden burst of energy. This sudden rush of sugary goodness is quickly converted into fast energy. The only problem is this energy doesn't last long and soon you're even hungrier than before. These sugar highs are horrible for the body. They deceive the body and allow it to think there is sufficient energy to sustain proper functions.

This in turn tricks your metabolism and it starts to derail its normal behavior.

The scientific stuff:

When sugar is consumed, certain areas of the brain are activated.

One, in particular, is the hippocampus. This part of the brain is linked with memory and inhibition.

The implications of this suggest that refined sugar directly affects your memory and inhibition and can interfere with short-term memory and learning.[2]

The hippocampus is impaired in a similar way when drugs are used.

Directly after sugar consumption, insulin is released, but more than the normal amount. This insulin overload gives the body a quick energy boost and is a huge health hazard.

This excess insulin directly leads to weight gain because the excess sugar needs to be immediately removed from the bloodstream and is stored in the cells as fat.

In short, your body isn't designed for these sugar rushes and tries to get rid of them the only way it knows how – by making you fat.

[1] Colantuoni C, Rada P, McCarthy J, Patten C, Avena NM, Chadeayne A, Hoebel BG..Evidence that intermittent, excessive sugar intake causes endogenous opioid dependence.Obes Res. 2002 Jun;10(6):478-88.

[2] Molteni R, Barnard RJ, Ying Z, Roberts CK, Gómez-Pinilla F.. A high-fat, refined sugar diet reduces hippocampal brain-derived neurotrophic factor, neuronal plasticity, and learning.Neuroscience. 2002;112(4):803-14.

4

Sugar Makes You Fat

You might be one of the many people reading this that share the common goal of losing weight and you need to realize that the consumption of sugar directly opposes this goal. Sugar has been researched, studied and researched again. All this research shows that sugar definitively contributes to obesity and unwanted weight gain.

In this section, we'll go over how sugar makes you gain weight, but first you need to know not all sugars are bad for us. For instance, glucose, the sugar found in your blood and in complex carbohydrates is the best kind of sugar. Your brain and every cell in your body can utilize and metabolize glucose.

Fruit, Fructose and High Fructose Corn Syrup

Fructose is easily the most misunderstood sugar. You read so much nowadays about the dangers of High Fructose Corn Syrup, and yet you are also told to get your regular servings of fruit in your diet. But doesn't fruit contain fructose?

Yes, one of the sugars found in fruit is fructose but there is a key difference between the fructose found in fruit and the high fructose corn syrup that resides in almost every processed/packaged food on the planet.

The fructose in fruit comes bundled with fiber, vitamins and minerals. The fiber slows down the absorption of the fructose allowing more of it to be converted into energy rather than into body fat.

Metabolic Disaster

Fructose can only be metabolized by the liver and from there it is usually converted into fat, bad cholesterol and/or uric acid. This differs from glucose, which is immediately distributed to and utilized by every cell in the body.

> *"Fructose does not stimulate insulin secretion or enhance leptin production. Because insulin and leptin act as key afferent signals in the regulation of food intake and body weight, this suggests that dietary fructose may contribute to increased energy intake and weight gain."* (Bray 2004)

High Fructose Corn Syrup $\left(HFCS \right)$

This stuff is in an abnormal amount of foods! Please check the labels of any processed food the next time you are in the grocery store.

> *"The increased use of HFCS in the United States mirrors the rapid increase in obesity."* (Bray 2004).

The body cannot process this type of sugar in large amounts. Excess amounts are directly stored as fat.

Repercussions of Excessive HFCS Consumption:

1. Excess fat (triglycerides) in the blood drastically elevates the risk for heart disease.

2. Fructose begins to deceive your regular appetite cues and leaves you still feeling hungry.

3. Having too much fructose in your diet may lead to insulin resistance, which in turn can lead to type 2 diabetes.

4. Consuming too much fructose may lead to a disease linked with obesity and diabetes called non-alcoholic fatty liver disease (NAFLD).

If you want to read more about HFCS, see this article by Eric Armstrong. For now, let's just agree, consuming this 'toxin' is not good for your health.

5

Sugar Causes Many Diseases

We began listing the many dire health consequences of sugar in the previous chapter. In addition to the maladies already mentioned, sugar is known to contribute to diabetes, weaken eyesight and to age your skin prematurely.

One huge problem with consuming too much sugar is that it provides no nutrients for the body. Too much sugar makes the brain crave more and more sugary foods.

A study[1] has shown by having two sugary drinks on a daily basis, you increase the risk of type 2 diabetes by about 25 percent! This is regardless of weight and overall health!

Women who drink more than two sugary drinks per day have a 40% higher risk of heart disease.[2]

Increased Consumption

To put things in perspective, about a hundred years ago, the average American consumed about 4 pounds of sugar per year.

Now the average American consumes about 180 pounds of sugar per year!

Just look at all the health problems people have nowadays. Like diabetes for instance, back then there were about 3 cases per 100,000 people living in the U.S. Now this number has risen to over 8,000 people per 100,000!

Need More Reasons?

If you still need more reasons to detox check out Nancy Appleton's list of 145 reasons to detox. Here's the link: 145 Reasons to Detox!

[1] Malik VS, Popkin BM, Bray GA, Després JP, Willett WC, Hu FB.. Sugar-sweetened beverages and risk of metabolic syndrome and type 2 diabetes: a meta-analysis. Diabetes Care. 2010 Nov;33(11):2477-83. doi: 10.2337/dc10-1079. Epub 2010 Aug 6.

[2] Fung TT, Malik V, Rexrode KM, Manson JE, Willett WC, Hu FB.Sweetened beverage consumption and risk of coronary heart disease in women.Am J Clin Nutr. 2009 Apr;89(4):1037-42. doi: 10.3945/ajcn.2008.27140. Epub 2009 Feb 11.

6

The Cleanse – What to Expect

To successfully complete a sugar cleanse, you need to know what to expect. Planning ahead and having a strong, positive mindset going in are vital in overcoming some of the obstacles you are going to face over the next 21 days.

For most people, you will be drastically changing your diet and some of the temporary side effects are not always…'enjoyable'. But not to worry, many other people have completed sugar cleanses before you and most of them will happily testify, the results are worth the effort.

If you need a little more incentive, just think back to the list of benefits from Chapter 1:

- weight loss
- increased energy
- increased stamina
- eliminate carvings for carbohydrates
- eliminate daily fatigue
- increased train of thought and concentration
- you will look better naked
- …and many more.

Negative Symptoms During the Cleanse

Some people experience negative symptoms during the first few days of their detox.

It is important you are aware of these symptoms, and that they do not last forever – they are just signals that your body is readjusting.

Symptoms resulting from a sugar detox can include:

- Fatigue
- Irritability
- Slight Nausea
- Minor Headaches
- Flu-like symptoms
- Cravings

As previously stated, these symptoms will pass, and the benefits of the detox will more than make up for a few days of discomfort.

Week One

- The beginning is always the most difficult part. Sugar cravings will be at their peak and you're going to want to give in. Don't worry and don't give in. After a few days these cravings should weaken and the longer you stay away from sugar the easier it becomes.
- The first week is when you will most likely experience some discomfort in the form of headaches, irritability, possible nausea and a host of other flu-like symptoms.
- Try to view these discomforts from a positive standpoint. These withdrawal symptoms are only temporary and the worse they are, the more your body is addicted to sugar and the more your body needs this detox.

Week Two

- Different people will feel difficult sugar withdrawal side effects. Some people may still be experiencing some discomfort from detox symptoms, while others will have already transitioned smoothly by this point.
- The most common discomfort in week two is a headache. If this happens be sure to drink plenty of water/green tea and these headaches will soon be a thing of the past.

Week Three

- Life should easy at this point. Sugar cravings should have stopped by now and you should have more energy than before. Your sleep will have also improved and you should feel like a new, healthier person!
- This final week is more about forming new healthy eating habits and improving your overall willpower in resisting future sugary temptations.

7

Shopping List - Good Foods to Eat

Food lists for Your Sugar Detox

Let's break it down further so you know exactly what you should and should not be eating to eliminate sugar from your diet.

For starters, here it the list of food to avoid while on a sugar detox:

- Bakery Products – Avoid all bakery products made from white flour.
- Carbohydrates – Avoid potatoes, white pasta, wheat pasta and white rice.
- Cereals/Grains – Avoid any cereal/grains not listed below, this includes pseudo grains like amaranth, buckwheat and quinoa.
- Dairy Products – Avoid all dairy; this includes cheese, yogurt and creamy sauces. **
- Fruit – Avoid all fruit not listed below.
- Legumes – Lentils, beans and peanuts.
- Liquids – Avoid alcohol, fruit juice and other sweetened beverages
- Diet drinks – Especially avoid these as they contain artificial sweeteners

- Sugar – Avoid all sugars, these include sucrose, fructose, high fructose corn syrup, cane sugar, honey, maple syrup and agave nectar.
- Other – MSG, trans fats, soy, hydrogenated oil, vinegar, fried foods.

So what can you eat?

Here's the list of approved foods while on a sugar detox:

- All Herbs and Spices.
- All Vegetables except starchy sources of carbohydrates like sweet potatoes and yams.***
- Wild and Brown Rice.
- Fruit: Avocado, Lemon, Lime, Tomatoes and all Berries.
- Meat: Organic turkey, chicken, beef, lamb. Wild salmon and other fish.
- Nuts and seeds.
- Oils: Coconut oil, Olive oil, Ghee and Butter.

** If you choose to drink dairy, consume only unpasteurized, full fat dairy.

*** Starchy carbohydrates like sweet potatoes, yams, etc. can be consumed in strict moderation.

Q. Am I eating a Paleolithic Diet?

A.   For those people familiar with the Paleo diet, yes the food selection of your sugar detox is similar to the meal plans of the Paleolithic diet. For those folks who aren't familiar with the Paleo diet, don't worry, it's not required prior knowledge to successfully complete your sugar detox.

Here is a shopping list you can take to the grocery store and load up with healthy, sugar detox friendly foods:

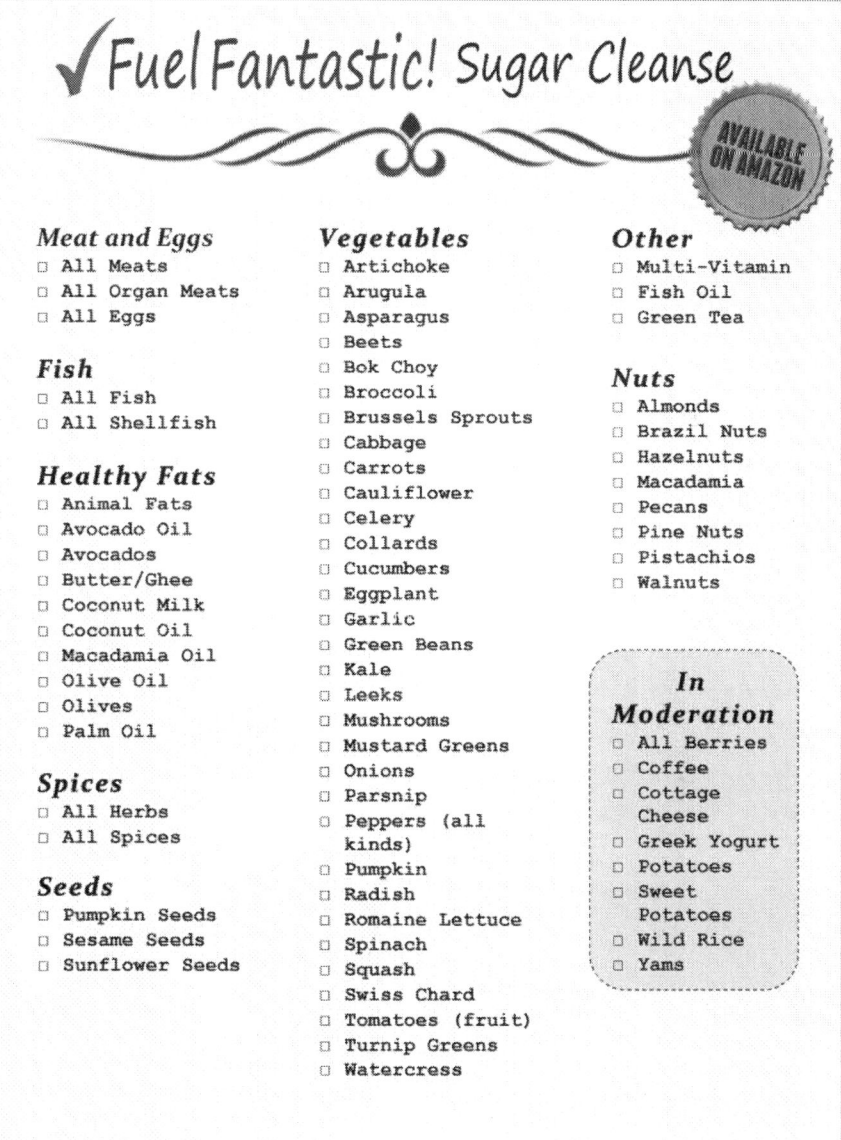

✓ Fuel Fantastic! Sugar Cleanse

AVAILABLE ON AMAZON

Meat and Eggs
- ☐ All Meats
- ☐ All Organ Meats
- ☐ All Eggs

Fish
- ☐ All Fish
- ☐ All Shellfish

Healthy Fats
- ☐ Animal Fats
- ☐ Avocado Oil
- ☐ Avocados
- ☐ Butter/Ghee
- ☐ Coconut Milk
- ☐ Coconut Oil
- ☐ Macadamia Oil
- ☐ Olive Oil
- ☐ Olives
- ☐ Palm Oil

Spices
- ☐ All Herbs
- ☐ All Spices

Seeds
- ☐ Pumpkin Seeds
- ☐ Sesame Seeds
- ☐ Sunflower Seeds

Vegetables
- ☐ Artichoke
- ☐ Arugula
- ☐ Asparagus
- ☐ Beets
- ☐ Bok Choy
- ☐ Broccoli
- ☐ Brussels Sprouts
- ☐ Cabbage
- ☐ Carrots
- ☐ Cauliflower
- ☐ Celery
- ☐ Collards
- ☐ Cucumbers
- ☐ Eggplant
- ☐ Garlic
- ☐ Green Beans
- ☐ Kale
- ☐ Leeks
- ☐ Mushrooms
- ☐ Mustard Greens
- ☐ Onions
- ☐ Parsnip
- ☐ Peppers (all kinds)
- ☐ Pumpkin
- ☐ Radish
- ☐ Romaine Lettuce
- ☐ Spinach
- ☐ Squash
- ☐ Swiss Chard
- ☐ Tomatoes (fruit)
- ☐ Turnip Greens
- ☐ Watercress

Other
- ☐ Multi-Vitamin
- ☐ Fish Oil
- ☐ Green Tea

Nuts
- ☐ Almonds
- ☐ Brazil Nuts
- ☐ Hazelnuts
- ☐ Macadamia
- ☐ Pecans
- ☐ Pine Nuts
- ☐ Pistachios
- ☐ Walnuts

In Moderation
- ☐ All Berries
- ☐ Coffee
- ☐ Cottage Cheese
- ☐ Greek Yogurt
- ☐ Potatoes
- ☐ Sweet Potatoes
- ☐ Wild Rice
- ☐ Yams

Link to printable download.

[http://bit.ly/YWo8nF]

8

How to Sugar Detox

The core concepts of cleansing your system of sugar are really quite basic. To achieve your goal, there are two different approaches you can follow. No matter which method you choose, your end goal is always going to be the same – removing sugar and it's addictions from your system.

Here are the two approaches to accomplish this goal:

    1. Weening Yourself Off Sugar Slowly

    2. Quitting Cold Turkey

Serious people always pick #2 and we're serious people, aren't we? Quitting sugar cold turkey is going to give you the best results.

When removing a band-aid, do you tear it off slowly (approach #1) or do you rip it off fast as possible? (approach #2)

How to Sugar Detox Cold Turkey

Here is how to detoxify your system with three simple guidelines:

- Only eat sugar-free foods from our approved shopping list
- Don't stop until you have completed 21 consecutive days.
- If you eat sugar, START OVER!

Pretty simple right? Well to tell you the truth, a sugar detox like any other detox is very easy in theory and much more difficult in practice.

Only Eat Sugar-free Foods

To make it easier for the more visually inclined, we have included a Sugar Detox Food Pyramid infographic.

SUGAR DETOX FOOD PYRAMID©
Approved Foods to Eat During Your Sugar Detox Diet

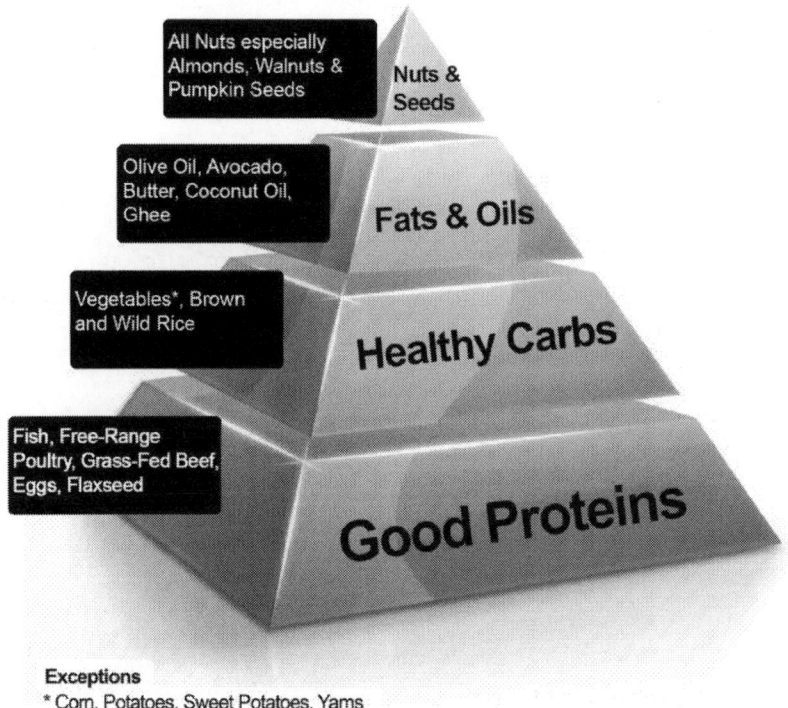

Exceptions
* Corn, Potatoes, Sweet Potatoes, Yams

Please Feel Free to Share this Infographic Courtesy of WeightLossNinja.org/Sugar-Detox

Please feel free to share this infographic with your family and friends. I recommend printing it out and putting it on the refrigerator door. [http://weightlossninja.org/sugar-cleanse-food-pyramid/]

PS. Corn is actually grain, not a vegetable.

To make the detox as easy as possible, you will be trying your best to maintain balanced blood glucose levels with no spikes and no dips.

How to maintain balanced blood glucose levels

Balancing blood 'glucose' levels is a breeze when you remove sugar from your diet because sugar (glucose) is the primarily reason your blood sugar spikes and dips on a daily basis. It is most definitely not the dietary fat you eat because dietary fat is metabolically inert. You can eat a stick of butter and your blood sugar doesn't even notice. Only proteins and carbohydrates effect your blood sugar with carbohydrates having the greatest impact. So once you remove sugar from your diet, you just need to do the following to maintain balanced blood sugar levels:

- Eat nutritionally balanced meals

All meals should include proteins, vegetables and healthy fats. That's it! So, what about snacking or eating smaller meals more frequently?

Myth: Eating Smaller Meals More Frequently

In our lifestyle diet plan guide (different book), we dive into this subject more deeply. There is no benefit to eating smaller meals more frequently. Please note, I said this is no benefit. If you already eat this way, there is no detriment to eating smaller meals more often either. But for people trying to lose weight, quite often they find it difficult to sustain this lifestyle with clean, healthy eating. With busy schedules and daily obligations, some of their smaller meals/snacks get filled with unhealthy food choices.

Most people associate snacks with their favorite carbohydrate filled meal replacements, like granola bars, protein bars, chips, chocolate bars, etc. To be successful, try and stay away form snacking and stick to only eating complete, balanced meals. If you need to snack in between meals, cook extra the night before and bring leftovers to eat as snacks.

If you accidentally eat sugar you have to start the detox over!

Sugar is very addictive so if you cheat and sneak a sugary trick once in awhile, you will fail in detoxing your system. There is no exceptions to this rule. If you eat sugar, you must start the detox over. Sorry. The same rules apply for everyone.

How Long Should You Detox For?

The length of your detox is entirely up to you and based on your individual situation with the word 'situation' being the key deciding factor on how long you perform the your sugar detox.

We will be covering two basic situations:

- First Timers – Sugar Detox Newbies
- Repeat Detoxers i.e. Biannual detox, etc.

First Timers

If you are a first time sugar detoxer and you think you can go the full three weeks – go for it! This is the most sure fire way to transition yourself into a healthier lifestyle.

Now don't use this next comment as an excuse to fail but most first timers are unable to go the full three weeks. So I present to you a challenge to be better than the majority and do the detox right the first time! (Please send me your success stories)

Repeat Detoxers

If you have completed a full sugar detox in the past, subsequent detoxes need only be two weeks in length. There is nothing wrong with going 3 or 4 weeks but you might find these extra weeks unnecessary.

*Note – If you are morbidly obese or have any medical conditions that might be a possible health concern, please seek medical advice before starting a sugar detox.

During and Following Your Detox

*Please make note of these important suggestions from some of our previous detoxers.

First, it may be wise to start your detox on a Friday evening/Saturday morning as you are likely to feel very tired for the first couple of days.

Second, avoid caffeine or switch to green tea, as it has amazing health properties and can act as a substitute for your morning hot drink.

It's advisable to take a multivitamin, particularly one with high levels of Vitamin C, as this can help detoxify the body.

Lastly, drinking water is really important. Staying hydrated can combat fatigue and assist with the detox.

After you have completed your 21 day detox, you can gradually add fruit and natural sweeteners like stevia (in moderation) back into your diet.

However, try to continue avoiding sucrose, high fructose corn syrup, wheat and soy.

9

Checklist for Success

There is no debating the fact that the first week of a sugar detox is by far the hardest week so being really prepared before you start is going to go a long way to your eventual success in completing the detox.

Complete as much of the following list as you can before you start the sugar detox:

- Write down your goals and motivation
- Remove all sugary temptations from the kitchen
- Stock the kitchen full of foods from the Shopping List.
- Plan and prepare the weeks meals
- Plan fun physical activities for the whole month
- Stay Hydrated
- Find your Support Group
- Food Journal (optional)

Goals and Motivation

- Setting your goals and reasons for completing this detox will inspire you during those times when your willpower starts to wane.

Remove Temptations

- Even people with the strongest willpower can easy fall victim to sugary temptations so do yourself a favor and cleanse the kitchen of all the food items that might derail your best intentions.

Stock the Kitchen

- One of the main focuses of this diet is to maintain balanced blood glucose levels. We want to remove the ups and downs that come with insulin spikes and dips. To accomplish this, we will want to make sure we have healthy food items on hand at all times and to only eat well balanced, complete meals throughout the day.

Plan and Prepare Meals

- Having pre-planned and prepared meals on hand really helps to keep you on track. Nothing is worse than being hungry and then having to wait while you prepare your dinner.

Plan Fun Activities

- The first week of a sugar detox is not the time to also try and start a new exercise regime. Especially one that you really are not truly interested in. Just staying active is all you need to distract your mind from the detox.

Stay Hydrated

- Many people mistaken thirst for hunger. One of the main withdrawal symptoms of a sugar detox are headaches and the best way to combat them is by staying hydrated.

Support Group

- One of the main reasons people fail in their diet efforts is because of outside influences. It is very important to make sure your family and friends are very supportive of your goals and efforts. (Read this article: Weight Loss Saboteurs)

10

Frequently Asked Questions

Q. Will I lose weight with a sugar detox?

A. Most people do lose weight during their 21 day sugar detox, but there are other factors to consider. Focus on your health first by practicing your new healthy eating habits and sustainable weight loss will be a natural by-product of this fun and active lifestyle.

Q. Do portion sizes matter?

A. For the most part, portion sizes don't matter Feel free to eat as many vegetables as you like. Make sure your plate is balanced with vegetables, healthy fats and protein. It is much more beneficial to eat a complete meal and be satiated, then to feel hungry after a meal and still craving carbohydrates.

Q. I've just started the sugar detox and I've had headaches for a few days, is this normal?

A. Don't worry. Headaches are common in the beginning. Your body is just adjusting to the lack of sugar and it is changing it's fuel source from carbohydrates to healthy fats. Be sure to drink plenty of water and eat when you're hungry. The headaches should clear up soon. Here is a great article explaining the low-carb flu in more detail.

[http://www.marksdailyapple.com/low-carb-flu/]

Q. Is coffee allowed?

A. Coffee is allowed, but remember no sugar. Drinking coffee might suppress appetite and then encourage it later. It depends on how you, as an individual react to caffeine. Just make sure coffee doesn't affect your sleep or your appetite. Some people choose to also detox from caffeine in unison with sugar. This can prove to be very difficult.

Q. Can I eat fruit during my detox?

A. Yes and No. Fruit contains fructose, which is a sugar. During the detox most fruits are best to be avoided, but after the detox is finished, we encourage you to start eating fruits again. The following fruits are encouraged in strict moderation during the sugar cleanse: Avocados, Lemons, Limes, Tomatoes and all Berries.

Q. What's the difference between the fructose found in fruit vs. the fructose found in processed foods?

A. Fruits are naturally packaged with fiber and nutrients that slow the absorption and digestion of the fructose. Whereas the fructose found in processed foods lack these important components and quite often overwhelm the liver.

11

Next Steps...What to do after your 1st Sugar Cleanse

Congratulations.

Most people never complete the full 21 days. No kidding. Many people don't even complete the 1st week, so pat yourself on the back. Three cheers for you; hip hip hooray, hip hip hooray, hip hip hooray.

Now what?

This is one of my friend's favorite sayings. At first I didn't really care for it but as time goes on I find it can be used in almost all aspects of life. You just completed a 21 day sugar detox, *now what?*

This next decision is entirely up to you but here are some suggestions for you to think about.

1. Start over and try to go for another 21 days!

2. Implement a new healthy lifestyle change, starting with your diet.

3. Write a short summary of your experiences and share them with our blog.

4. All of the above.

Let's Do It Again!

Q. Why on Earth would I want to try another 21 day sugar detox?

A. For most people, 21 days is not enough time to form a habit or to completely break free of their addictions to sugar. By starting another detox immediately, you will be reinforcing your resolve towards sugar's ills and forming new healthy eating habits.

Implement a Healthy Lifestyle Change

This is the preferred option. Start a new diet, join the gym, buy a rowing machine, join a hiking club, train for a 10 kilometer run.

The possibilities are endless. Talk hold of your new found energy and cravings for healthy food and propel yourself into a more active lifestyle, filled with yummy foods, new friends and lots of fun, physical activities.

Share Your Experiences

The best motivation usually comes from watching someone else complete their goals. So here is the perfect opportunity to share your experiences and inspire others to follow in your footsteps to a fun, healthy, new lifestyle.

Send us your story. We'd love to share your story on our blog or on one of our Facebook pages.

Go here and fill out our contact form.

[http://bit.ly/W9rHlZ]

Thank You

We hope you enjoyed the Fuel Fantastic Sugar Cleanse brought to you by the authors of Weight Loss Ninja.

If your future goals include losing weight, eating clean and getting lean, we hope you will become a regular participant at our blog.

By first detoxing your system of sugar, you will be able to be much more successful in transitioning yourself into a healthier and happier lifestyle.

We want to hear you feedback and your detox success stories, so please email us at: contact@weightlossninja.org

If think someone you know might benefit from this guide, please help spread the awareness and feel free to share this link with them.

http://weightlossninja.org

Thanks for your support.

- Kelly Fitzsimmons -

Bonus Chapter: Stevia - Nature's Sugar Substitute

Stevia's scientific name is Stevia Rebaudiana, and in addition to 'stevia' is also called sweetleaf and sugarleaf.

The genus is a large collection, with over two hundred species of plants from the sunflower family.

Where is Stevia Produced?

Stevia is native to tropics and subtropics of South and Central America. Some species are also found in certain areas of North America, such as Texas and Arizona for example. The plant has been grown by indigenous groups in South America for over 1500 years.

What is Stevia Used For?

Stevia is used as a sugar substitute and sweetener. Fresh stevia leaves have over thirty times the sweetness of sucrose and their taste has a slower onset and duration.

Although the plant has been used by indigenous people for over a thousand years, it was only introduced to Western science in 1899, by a Swiss botanist. In 1931, the glycosides which give the plant its sweet taste were isolated by French chemists and they were named rebaudioside and stevioside. These glycosides are almost 300 times as sweet as sucrose and non-fermentable.

In addition, they are pH and heat stable.

These highly sweet glycosides can have a bitter aftertaste.

Of them, rebaudioside A is the least bitter and as such is often the target of commercial production. This involves extracting the rebaudioside from dried stevia leaves, first by water extraction and then by crystallization which separates the glycoside molecules.

The result is pure rebaudioside A.

The tongue reacts to the glucose in the glycosides. As rebaudiosides have more glucose than steviosides, thus they taste sweeter to us. Glycosides also contain aglycones, non-sugar substances, and these can activate some of the tongue's bitter receptors.

After ingesting rebaudioside, it is metabolized into stevioside which in turn is broken down into steviol and glucose. The glucose is not absorbed into the blood stream but is used by the bacteria in our gut, and steviol is simply passed from the digestive system as waste.

Commercial Usage

Stevia extracts, steviol glycosides, were first made commercially available by a Japanese company in the early 1970s.

These can have up to 300 times the sweetness of sugar. This combined with the fact that stevia has no measurable effect on blood glucose, mean that stevia has drawn wide interest as a natural alternative to sugar for people on sugar and carbohydrate controlled diets.

Japan leads the way when it comes to the use of stevia as a sweetener with around 40% of their sweetener market being made up of stevia products.

In Japan, stevia is found in soft drinks and food, as well as being available for table use. This reliance on stevia developed as a result of concerns over other sweeteners, e.g. saccharin, being carcinogenic.

Stevia is grown and used in food products in many East Asian countries, as well as in much of South America. It's usage in America and the EU is a recent development due to previous concerns over safety (see next section).

In the States, Coca-Cola has developed a stevia-derived sweetener called rebiana, marketed as Truvia, which was approved as a food additive in 2008. With stevia also being approved in the EU in 2011, we're sure to see it becoming more widely available over the next few years.

It is safe?

Although widely available in parts of Asia and South America for more than thirty years, there has been some controversy over stevia's usage in the USA and the EU.

A study[1] in the 1980s reported that steviol acted as a mutagen in a rat's liver. The findings were criticized as flawed and further studies[2] went on to find that steviol did not produce harmful effects.

The World Health Organization performed their own investigation[3] of stevioside and rebaudioside finding both of them to be non-toxic. They went on to find no evidence of carcinogenic properties, something that has been a concern for other sweeteners, and noted the possible benefits of stevia for those with hypertension and type-2 diabetes (see next section).

The World Health Organization conducted a follow-up study[4] which approves the daily intake of steviol glycoside at a maximum of 4mg/kg body weight. This means that all food and beverages containing stevia extracts are subject to restriction. The American Food Standards Agency recognized rebaudioside A as safe in 2009.

Secondary Health Benefits of Stevia

The primary usage for stevia is as an alternative to sugar. However, some studies have found some further interesting benefits.

For example, a study[5] conducted in 2009, found that stevioside has anti-imflammatory, anti-tumour, anti-hypertensive, anti-diarrheal and antihyperglycemic properties.

Stevia's effect on diabetes has also been widely investigated. In rats, stevia has been shown to improve sensitivity to insulin.[6]

Stevia can also revitalize the beta cells of the pancreas and may also promote insulin production.

Eating stevia before meals can reduce insulin levels following the meal when compared to other sweeteners. A study in 2011[7] concluded that stevia would therefore benefit diabetic individuals.

Where to Buy Stevia and How to Use It

With evidence stacking up in favor of stevia as a viable alternative to sugar, you'll probably want to know where you can get hold of some. There are a multitude of websites now selling stevia products.

You can buy stevia in liquid, powder and tablet form. The tablets and liquid forms are easily dissolved in drinks while the powder is best used in cooking.

A 25 gram shaker of stevia powder contains 1000 servings meaning 1/3 teaspoon is about the equivalent of one cup of sugar.

Final Words

Marketers of stevia tout it as a 'natural' alternative to sugar, but unless you're using the actual plants this isn't strictly true.

However, when you consider stevia extracts in comparison to the aspartame and saccharin products that are also widely available, and the controversy that often surrounds these additives, I think you'll agree that stevia makes for a pretty sweet alternative.

[1] Pezzuto JM, Compadre CM, Swanson SM, Nanayakkara D, Kinghorn AD (April 1985)."Metabolically activated steviol, the aglycone of stevioside, is mutagenic". *Proc. Natl. Acad. Sci. U.S.A.* 82 (8): 2478–82

[2] Geuns JM (2003). "Stevioside". *Phytochemistry* 64 (5): 913–21.

[3] Benford, D.J.; DiNovi, M., Schlatter, J. (2006). "Safety Evaluation of Certain Food Additives: Steviol Glycosides" *WHO Food Additives Series* (World Health Organization Joint FAO/WHO Expert Committee on Food Additives (JECFA)) 54: 140

[4] Joint FAO/WHO Expert Committee on food additives, Sixty-ninth Meeting. World Health Organization. 4 July 2008

[5] Chatsudthipong, V.; Muanprasat, C. (Jan 2009). "Stevioside and related compounds: therapeutic benefits beyond sweetness.". *Pharmacol Ther* 121 (1): 41–54

[6] Lailerd N, Saengsirisuwan V, Sloniger JA, Toskulkao C, Henriksen EJ (January 2004)."Effects of stevioside on glucose transport activity in insulin-sensitive and insulin-resistant rat skeletal muscle". *Metab. Clin. Exp.* 53 (1): 101–7

[7] Goyal, SK.; Samsher, RK.; Goyal. (Feb 2010). "Stevia (Stevia rebaudiana) a bio-sweetener: a review". *Int J Food Sci Nutr* 61 (1): 1–10

Bonus Chapter: The Dangers of Glycation

One of the major ways that sugar disrupts our health is through a process called glycation.

Glycation happens when a sugar molecule attaches itself to a lipid or protein molecule and in doing so, changes healthy, flexible tissue into hard and rigid tissue. This tough glycated tissue causes the skin to become wrinkled and also causes internal damage to organs that need flexible tissue to stay healthy.

Glycated tissue is also very dangerous because it produces toxic compounds called Advanced Glycation End-products (AGEs).

These molecules go by a highly appropriate acronym, because they are detrimental to our bodies and they also assist in rapidly advancing the aging process.

AGEs are the most toxic product of glycation and you must make it a priority focus to reduce them in your diet.

How are AGEs formed?

In a diet with a healthy, low sugar intake, proteins and sugars can interact without damaging the body. But when the body takes in too much sugar, excess sugars can attach themselves to protein molecules, which changes how these proteins function, creating a non-functioning glycated protein molecule: an **AGE**.

AGEs can also be found in some of the foods we eat.

Not only associated with sugar, AGEs are present in many processed foods and foods that are cooked over high temperatures. Many processed or pre-prepared foods contain AGEs because they are the very compounds which give food that tasty, irresistible aspect we love so much.

Think about the taste, smell and appearance of fried chicken, a grilled bacon cheeseburger, corn chips, or fresh cookies. These foods are highly appealing, and hard to stop eating even after your body might be full. Food manufacturers use processes like browning and caramelization to make foods delicious, but these processes add tons of AGEs into the foods we eat.

Why are AGEs toxic?

AGEs are oxidants that corrode our body the same way that rust corrodes metal.

When food AGEs are consumed in small amounts, the body is able to counter their effects with antioxidants. But excess AGE consumption and/or the production of AGEs through glycation can overwhelm the naturally produced antioxidants we consume via our fruit and vegetable intake. Once these protective resources are depleted, AGEs go to work damaging major vital organs and ruthlessly hastening the aging process.

The body reacts to AGEs as it would to any infection, by creating low level inflammation (a person with an infection may experience a fever, indicating inflammation, which will pass with the infection.) But as AGEs pile up in the body, inflammation becomes chronic. This prolonged inflammation slowly but surely goes on to damage every organ in the body.

How does glycation contribute to aging?

Glycation directly hastens the aging process in nearly every organ, including the skin, heart, brain, eyes and pancreas (organs where flexibility is especially vital.) The tough, inflexible tissue produced by glycation is the enemy of youthful skin and organs, making it difficult for the body to function properly. But the AGEs created by glycation are the biggest threat to health and vitality.

AGEs produce small molecules called reactive oxygen species (ROS) that cause major tissue damage and oxidation. To make matters worse, the reactive oxygen species help to create even more AGEs in the body, setting up a vicious cycle that accelerates the aging process.

AGEs also create chemical bridges between proteins, making joints and tendons stiffer and thicker as the body ages. But it's not only the skin and joints that are involved; hardened arteries, cataracts in the eyes and damaged heart and kidneys are other byproducts of the glycation process. (Sorry for all the doom and gloom, I'm just delivering a needed message.)

A high level of AGEs in the blood guarantees high AGEs in the skin as well causing the skin to quickly lose its youthful appearance and become tough, dry and wrinkled.

AGEs also make it more difficult for wounds to heal increasing the likelihood they become infected and form scars. They are also major contributors to cardiovascular disease, hypertension, stroke, dementia, kidney disease and diabetes.

And the scary truth is that the toxic effect of AGEs is hard at work long before there is any sign of disease in the body.

How can glycation be reduced?

The good news after all of this is that while glycation cannot currently be reversed, it can be significantly reduced and prevented through changes to diet and lifestyle.

The toxic effects of glycation are so prevalent today, with all the available highly processed foods that are packed with sugars and AGEs. It's so important to make a commitment to health and take the steps toward reducing aging and maintaining health, balance and vitality in your own body.

Here are some tips for protecting yourself from AGEs and the toxic effects of glycation:

- **Reduce sugar intake** – It is widely known that sugar is a major cause of degenerative diseases, but somehow its consumption continues to increase each year. Glycation feeds on sugar, and sugar is hidden in processed foods where you might not expect it: in condiments and sauces, crackers, cereals, dairy products, beverages, almost anything that comes in a box or package.

- **Limit carbohydrates** – The body reacts to carbohydrates the same way that is reacts to simple sugars, so an overabundance will cause glycation and AGEs just like sugar does. Reduce your intake of breads, pasta and wheat.

- **Eliminate high fructose corn syrup** - Scan labels for this ingredient and avoid it at all costs.

- **Eat a balanced diet of vegetables, fats and protein** – Choosing foods which keep blood sugar levels stable limits glycation in the body. Some good sources for fats and protein include eggs, meat, nuts, seeds and healthy oils like coconut, olive and avocado oil.

- **Eat vegetables raw, boiled or steamed, and cook meats low and slow** – AGEs can be produced when foods are cooked at high temperatures, so avoid frying, grilling and searing foods whenever possible. Water also prevents sugars from binding to protein molecules, so cooking with water or steam helps prevent glycation.

- **Choose water over sugary beverages** - Soft drinks and juices are one of the major sources of excess sugar in many people's diets, a problem that can easily be corrected by simply drinking water! Water replaces these sugary contributors to AGEs, while providing a whole host of other health benefits to the body.
- **Try supplements** - While there is currently no known way to reverse glycation, there are supplements that have been shown to inhibit the process and protect the body. **Carnosine** is has been shown to protect against AGEs and rejuvenate aging skin tissue. Pyridoxamine, a form of Vitamin B6, is also a natural inhibitor in the formation of AGEs.

The most important things to remember when setting out to protect your body from glycation are:

- Avoiding foods that are high in AGEs.
- Avoiding consumption of excess sugar and carbohydrates.
- Using cooking methods and temperatures which prevent the formation of new AGEs. (keep cooking temperatures under 110 Celsius)

By keeping these three key principles in mind, along with the tips described above, you will be well on your way to protecting your body from the devastating aging effects of glycation.

It's never easy to revamp your diet and lifestyle, especially in today's society where processed foods and tasty options are abundant around every tempting corner. So rather than striving for perfection, focus instead on maintaining a healthy balance by vegetables, healthy proteins and fats in your diet.

Your body is well and able to deal with a controlled amount of AGEs as long as they do not overload your system, and you consume enough antioxidants to counter their effects.

Bonus Chapter: Top 10 Foods Surprisingly High in Sugar

Here is our top 10 list of foods that we think are surprisingly high in sugar:

1. Granola Bars

Advertising gives granola bars an illusion of being a healthy snack.

Slim, fit people are often pictured enjoying a granola bar after a hike in nature or a hard workout.

Contrary to this image, granola bars contain a lot of sugar.

In fact, if you look at the ingredient list on a granola bar, sugar is likely to be in the top 5, making it nutritionally similar to a candy bar.

Tip: Make your own:

Trail mix – Stir in a combination of nuts, muesli, unsweetened dried fruit, and dark chocolate. Easy as pie.

Peanut Butter Granola Bars

Ingredients:

- 1 cup peanut butter
- 1 cup tahini
- 2 cups honey
- 1 tsp sea salt

Blend above ingredients together completely.

- 1 cup sesame seeds
- 1 cup almond (coarsely chopped)
- 2 cups coconut
- 2 cups sunflower seeds
- 2 cups dark chocolate chips
- 2 cups rolled oats (toasted and cooled)

  1. Blend remaining ingredients into previous mixture taking care not to over mix.

  2. Press dough firmly and evenly in greased pan.

  3. Bake at 350 degrees.

  4. Cook on bottom shelf for 15 minutes, spin, and move to the middle rack for and additional 8 minutes.

  5. Do not overcook, they brown easily.

  6. Bars should be evenly brown when finished. Remove from oven, cool, cut, and enjoy.

2. Tomato Sauce

One cup of tomato sauce can contain over 20 grams of sugar.

Due to the fact that most people eat tomato sauce on top of a mound of pasta, an already high source of carbohydrates, this can be an extreme sugar overload.

Tip: Tomato sauce can easily be made from scratch using tomato paste, fresh, or canned tomatoes.

Use caramelized onions or carrots to sweeten the sauce and mask the acidity of the tomatoes.

3. Fruit Juices

Although "100 percent juice" and "all natural" sound healthier than their competitors, chances are they are still packed with sugar.

It is true that a portion of this sugar naturally is from the fruit itself, however consuming the fruit whole will provide the added fiber intake that is missing in its liquid form.

Tip: If you have your own juicer, use it!

4. Yogurt

Yogurt is always being praised as one of the healthiest of foods as it boosts metabolism and increases immunity to illnesses.

However some varieties actually aid in pushing your daily intake of sugar to the limits.

A heaping 27 grams of sugar is in a 6 ounce container of Yoplait flavored yogurt.

When in doubt, it is always best to pick either plain or Greek yogurt and still make sure to check the label before buying.

Tip: Use the sweet flavor of blueberries to liven up plain yogurt.

5. Muffins

I agree muffins are healthier than opting for a doughnut to compliment a morning cup of coffee but they also contain a good deal of sugar. Even store/bakery bought bran muffins have around 20 grams of sugar. To avoid this I suggest making your own, there are several recipes that do not require sugar at all and taste the same.

Tip: To sweeten up bland tasting bran muffins add bananas, blueberries, raspberries, mangos...up to you!

6. Canned Fruit

A fair amount of canned fruit is packaged in a sugary syrup which combined with the fruit itself is enough to send one into sugar overload.

Even light syrup has a whopping 32 grams of sugar per one cup serving.

Opt for the fruit canned in natural fruit juice or just eat the real deal.

Tip: Buy fresh fruit, pre-cut, and store in the refrigerator. This way it'll always be on hand, absent of added sugar.

7. Cereal

For many people, a bowl of cereal is the first meal of the day, which is advertised as being beneficial to one's health because of the fiber. Any benefit derived from this boost in fiber is quickly negated if the bowl of cereal is pack full of processed sugar.

Claims of being healthy often masks this detail, even select wholesome granola based cereals contain as much as 13 grams of sugar per serving.

To avoid this read nutrition labels, you may be surprised by the difference.

Tip: Purchase basic granola or muesli in the bulk section and make your own breakfast cereal. This way you can dodge sneaky sugar filled cereals and dress it up to your preference.

Yogurt, fresh fruit, honey....yum!

8. Vitamin Water

Vitamin water contains essential vitamins, minerals and gives you a boost of energy.

However, don't be so easily deceived, that extra energy after taking the last drink is a sugar high incognito.

A bottle of Snapple's Antioxidant Water or Glaceau's Vitamin Water holds more than 30 grams of sugar in a 20-ounce bottle.

You're better off drinking regular water and taking vitamins to avoid this extra sugar intake. Also, it will be much cheaper in the long run.

Tip: If you crave a little flavor in your water infuse it with lemon, lime or cucumbers.

9. Fat Free Salad Dressings

Fat free = healthy. Not necessarily and when it comes to salad dressings most companies pump loads of sugar into their products to give them an appetizing taste. Check labels to find a healthy compromise of fat and sugar or make your own dressing.

Tip: Simple Balsamic Vinaigrette Recipe

Ingredients:

- 1/4 cup balsamic vinegar
- 1 tsp minced garlic
- 1/2 tsp freshly ground pepper
- 1/2 tsp salt
- 3/4 cup olive oil

    1. Combine vinegar, garlic, pepper, salt and whisk together blending completely.

    2. Beat in olive oil in small amounts, continuing to whisk (or pour all ingredients in a seal tight screw top container and shake.)

*If you are not consuming the dressing right away, cover and refrigerate. Whisk or shake before reuse.

10. Smoothies

Fruit smoothies can be super healthy if prepared in a wholesome fashion. Be aware of the sugar content of commercially bought smoothies.

Even those prepared with fresh fruit at a restaurant or shop may have added sugar. To dodge this make your smoothies at home where you have complete control over the ingredients.

Tip: Avocado Smoothie

Ingredients:

- 1 ripe avocado
- 1 cup almond milk
- 1/2 cup yogurt
- 3 tablespoons honey

Combine all the ingredients in a blender and mix until smooth.

Final Thoughts

The above foods are only a limited list of the most surprising foods that contain high levels of sugar and unfortunately it most definitely doesn't stop there. As mindful consumers, we should all become more knowledgeable about the food we are feeding our bodies.

Also whenever possible always try to eat food that is as close to it's original form as possible. Your body and wallet will thank you.

Sources

• Avena N., et al. (2007). Evidence for sugar addiction: Behavioral and neurochemical effects of intermittent, excessive sugar intake. Neuroscience & Biobehavioral Reviews. 32: 1 . 20–39.

• Bray, G.A. (2008). Fructose: should we worry? International Journal of Obesity. 32, S127-S131.

• Bray, G.A., et al. (2004). Consumption of high-fructose corn syrup in beverages may play a role in the epidemic of obesity. American Journal of Clinical Nutrition. 79, 4, 537-543.

• Colantuoni, C., et al. (2001). Evidence That Intermittent, Excessive Sugar Intake Causes Endogenous Opioid Dependence. Obesity Research. 10, 478–488.

• Francis, H.M., Stevenson, R.J. (2011). Higher reported saturated fat and refined sugar intake is associated with reduced hippocampal-dependent memory and sensitivity to interoceptive signals. Behav Neurosci. 125(6):943-55.

• Molteni, R., et al. (2002). A high-fat, refined sugar diet reduces hippocampal brain-derived neurotrophic factor, neuronal plasticity, and learning. Neuroscience. 112: 4. 803–814.

Other Books By Kelly Fitzsimmons

Fuel Fantastic Diet That Works

You need to make this lifestyle change, today!

Fuel Fantastic will forever change your mindset towards nutrition, food, health and dietary advice.

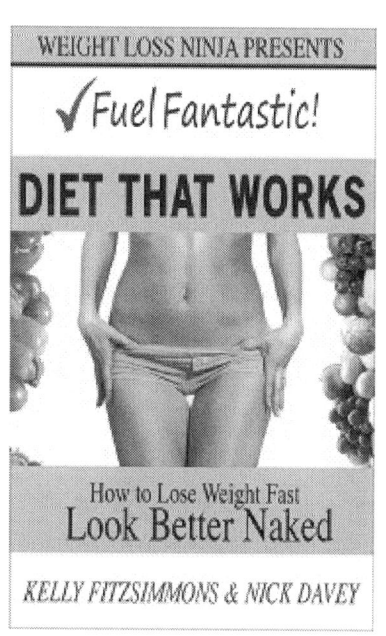

Utilizing its long-term, evidence based, sustainable approach, you will get the results you want and you will quickly learn how to live a healthier lifestyle.

Fuel Fantastic is the definitive guide to losing weight, eating clean and getting lean... but it also goes way beyond just being a diet book.

How to Lose Weight Fast and Look Better Naked!

Using Fuel Fantastic, you will be able to heal your metabolism so it functions properly and runs faster than it ever has before.

The many other benefits you can immediately expect to start realizing as soon as you start your new lifestyle are:

- Hunger carvings are quickly eliminated
- Counting calories is not needed
- Energy and vitality is increased in mere days
- You start craving healthy foods

- You wake up each day refreshed ready to take on the world
- Your body bursts through weight loss plateaus
- You get to eat bacon and eggs!
- You will look better naked
- Nobody needs to know you're on a diet, because you not!

Inside Fuel Fantastic, you will quickly discover the key dietary myths that have prevented you from losing weight for all these years.

We've solved all the problems most diets fail to address and make it easy for our dieters to keep doing what they want to be doing; losing weight while living a normal lifestyle.

Download your copy now and Let's Fuel Fantastic

4278448R00043

Printed in Great Britain
by Amazon.co.uk, Ltd.,
Marston Gate.